How to Prepare and Use Herbal Remedies for Home Health Care: Herbs for Common Illnesses.

Mary S. Nordin

Table of contents

Understanding Herbs

Chapter 1

Herbal medicine (also called **herbalism**) is the study of pharmacognosy and the use of medicinal plants. The scope of herbal medicine sometimes include fungal and bee products, as well as minerals, shells and certain animal parts.

Herbs are the most wonderfully diverse and useful plants, coming in all shapes, sizes and textures, colours and perfumes. Their aromatic leaves and scented flowers can be enjoyed by all, making them the most generous of plants.

But what is a Herb?

We believe that 'all useful plants are herbs'.
The **Oxford English Dictionary** defines them as 'any

plant with leaves, seeds, or flowers used for flavouring, food, medicine, or perfume.'

The **RHS** describes Herbs as *'versatile garden plants. Pretty enough to grow in an ornamental border, many will also thrive in containers. You can also grow tender herbs, such as basil, indoors or in a greenhouse.'*

Finally, **Wikipedia**, states that herbs are *'plants with savoury or aromatic properties that are used for flavouring and garnishing food, medicinal purposes, or for fragrances'*.

In conclusion, we prefer our definition, if it is useful, it is most probably a herb.

How are Herbs named?

Plants are assigned to a family and their name is comprised of their genus and botanical name. This allows horticulturists, and anyone interested in plants, around the world to understand the plants they are looking at and determine their uses and how to maintain and grow them.

Here are some basic tips for understanding Latin and plant names:

- **'*x*'** indicates a hybrid. Some species, when grown together in the wild or in cultivation are found to interbreed and form hybrids. These rarely set viable seed.
- ***vulgare*** this is the common variety of herb
- ***officinalis*** this indicates that it was officially used by the ancient apothecaries
- ***AGM*** these initials after the botanical name indicate that the plant has been awarded the RHS' Award of Garden Merit.

An example of a Hybrid mint is **Mentha x piperita (Peppermint),** which in the past has been known as Menta d'Angletterre, Mentha anglais, pfefferminze and Englisheminze. The hybridisation (x) to create this mint was between water mint, *Mentha aquatica* and spearmint, *Mentha spicata*.

We understand that Herbs are any useful plants and that using Latin names allows herb enthusiasts to understand what they are looking at.

What are the differences between annual, biennial and perennial herbs?

Annual, biennial and perennial are some of the common names for the describing the life evolution or stages of herbs. The main terms are:

- **Annual herbs**- a plant that lives for just one season.
- **Biennial herbs**- a plant that produces leaves in the first season and flowers in the second year then produces seed and dies.
- **Perennial herbs**- a plant that lives for a number of seasons, most flower annually once established.

What are the main herb families?

The next thing to consider is the plant families and how different species actually relate to one another (like your cousins). When reading a plant name, the family name is easily recognised as it ends in -aceae. The main herb families are listed below,

ALLIACEAE HERB FAMILY

This family includes herbaceous monocot plants that are generally perennial but not evergreen. Most are native to dry or moderately moist regions and other open areas. The family includes bulb or corm-forming plants as well as plants without bulbs or corms. Leaves may be round, flat, or angular in cross section and are alternately or spirally arranged. The leaves of most species in the Alliaceae are aromatic, frequently smelling like onion. Flowers are generally organised into ball-or umbel-shaped clusters. Herbs of the Allium family such as ***Allium schoenoprasum*** (Chives) and ***Allium sativum*** (Garlic) are well known examples of this

APIACEAE HERB FAMILY

This family is more commonly known as the celery, carrot or parsley family, or simply as umbellifer. The herbs in this family are flavourful and aromatic and include ***Foeniculum vulgare*** (Fennel),

Levisticum officinale (Lovage), *Petroselinum crispum* (Parsley) and *Anthriscus cerefolium* (Chervil). Their leaves are of variable size and alternately arranged, or with the upper leaves becoming nearly opposite. Plants in this family have flowers that nearly always aggregated in terminal umbels.

ASTERACEAE HERB FAMILY

This family is commonly referred to as the daisy family and mostly contains herbaceous herbs that have taproots. For example, *Calendula Officinalis* (Pot Marigold), *Echinacea* (Cone Flowers) and *Achillea millefolium* (Yarrow). This family is used in herbal infusions, herbal medicines and salads. Nearly all members bear their flowers in dense heads in what appears to be a single flower when it is actually a cluster of much smaller flowers. The name Asteraceae comes from the type genus Aster that is Ancient Greek for star and refers to the star-like form of the flower.

BRASSICACEA HERB FAMILY

Brassicaceae is an economically important family of flowering plants commonly known as the mustards, the crucifers or the cabbage family. They are comprise of annuals, biennials, perennials and herbaceous plants and can be found growing throughout the world. The important vegetables in this family include, cabbage, broccoli, Brussel sprouts, kale and radish to name a few.

LAMIACEAE HERB FAMILY

One of the largest families that is commonly called the mint or dead-nettle family. It includes the most widely used culinary herbs, such as, *Origanum*(Oregano), Hyssopus (Hyssop), *Lavandula* (Lavender), *Mentha*

(Mint) and *Thymus* (Thyme). Most members of the family are perennial or annual herbs with square stems. The leaves are typically simple and oppositely arranged; most are fragrant and contain volatile oils. These herbs are readily propagated by stem cuttings.

MYRTACEAE HERB FAMILY

This amazing family can be found growing throughout the world in the tropics, subtropics and Mediterranean. It contains, trees and shrubs, many of which are important herbs and spices including Syzygium aromaticum, Cloves and Pimenta dioica, All spice. The family takes its name from the shrub Myrtus which is found near the Mediterranean

Chapter 2
The Art of Making Herbal Hemedies

Herbs have been used for their medicinal properties for thousands of years, and today, more and more people are rediscovering the power of herbs for health and wellness. Whether you're a seasoned herb gardener or just starting out, growing and using herbs for medicinal purposes can be a rewarding and satisfying experience.

We'll explore the various aspects of growing and using herbs for medicinal purposes, including tips on growing and harvesting herbs, making herbal remedies, and using herbs in everyday life.

The first step to using herbs for medicinal purposes is to grow them yourself or purchase them from a reputable source. When growing herbs, it's important to choose the right location, soil, and watering regime to ensure the plants are healthy and vigorous. Some common herbs used for medicinal purposes include:

• Calendula for skin health
• Echinacea for boosting the immune system
• Lavender for relaxation and stress relief
• Peppermint for digestive health

Once you have your herbs, it's time to learn about the various ways to use them for medicinal purposes, including:

• Making herbal teas
• Creating herbal tinctures and extracts
• Infusing oils and salves
• Adding herbs to food and drinks

Making Herbal Remedies

One of the most popular ways to use herbs for medicinal purposes is to make herbal remedies, such as teas, tinctures, and infusions. When making herbal remedies, it's important to follow proper dosing guidelines and seek the advice of a healthcare professional if necessary.

For example, a simple herbal tea can be made by steeping dried or fresh herbs in boiling water for several minutes. Herbal tinctures can be made by soaking herbs in alcohol or glycerin for several weeks, and extracts can be made by soaking herbs in hot water or oil to extract the medicinal properties.

Herbs can also be used in everyday life to support health and wellness, such as:

• Adding herbs to your cooking and baking for added flavor and health benefits
• Making herbal bath teas for relaxation and stress relief
• Using herbal sprays for cleaning and freshening the air
• Adding herbs to skincare products for added benefits

Herbs are not just for medicinal purposes –
they can also be used in a variety of ways to
enhance your daily life and promote health
and wellness.

In conclusion, growing and using herbs for
medicinal purposes can be a rewarding and
satisfying experience. Whether you're
making herbal remedies, using herbs in
everyday life, or simply enjoying the beauty
of a herb garden, herbs can play a valuable
role in promoting health and wellness. So,
why not get started today and explore the
world of herbal medicine.

HERBAL MEDICINE: A GROWING FIELD WITH A LONG TRADITION

Traditional medicine is "the
knowledge, skills and practices based
on the theories, beliefs and experiences
indigenous to different cultures, used
in the maintenance of health and in the
prevention, diagnosis, improvement or

treatment of physical and mental illness" (World Health Organization)

There are many different systems of traditional medicine, and the philosophy and practices of each are influenced by the prevailing conditions, environment, and geographic area within which it first evolved (WHO 2005), however, a common philosophy is a holistic approach to life, equilibrium of the mind, body, and the environment, and an emphasis on health rather than on disease. Generally, the focus is on the overall condition of the individual, rather than on the particular ailment or disease from which the patient is suffering, and the use of herbs is a core part of all systems of traditional medicine.

Traditional Chinese medicine (TCM) is an important example of how ancient and accumulated knowledge is applied in a holistic approach in present day health care. TCM has a history of more than 3000 years (Xutian, Zhang, and Louise 2009). The book *The Devine Farmer's Classic of Herbalism* was compiled about 2000 years ago in China and is the oldest known herbal text in the world, though the accumulated and methodically collected information on herbs has been developed into various herbal pharmacopoeias and many monographs on individual herbs exist.

Diagnosis and treatment are based on a holistic view of the patient and the patient's symptoms, expressed in terms of the balance of yin and yang. Yin represents the earth, cold, and femininity, whereas yang represents the sky, heat, and masculinity. The actions of yin and yang influence the interactions of the five elements composing the universe: metal, wood, water, fire, and earth. TCM practitioners seek to control the yin and yang levels through 12 meridians, which bring and channel energy (Qi) through the body. TCM is a growing practice around the world and is used for promoting health as well as for preventing and curing diseases.

Over the past 100 years, the development and mass production of chemically synthesized drugs have revolutionized health care in most parts of the word. However, large sections of the population in developing countries still rely on traditional practitioners and herbal medicines for their primary care. In Africa up to 90% and in India 70% of the population depend on traditional medicine to help meet their health care needs. In China, traditional medicine accounts for around 40% of all health care delivered and more than 90% of general hospitals in China have units for traditional medicine (WHO 2005). However, use of traditional medicine is not limited to developing countries, and during the past two decades public interest in natural therapies has increased greatly in industrialized countries, with expanding use of ethnobotanicals. In the United States, in 2007, about 38% of adults and 12% of children were using some form of traditional medicine (Ernst, Schmidt, and Wider 2005; Barnes, Bloom, and Nahin 2008). According to a survey by the National Center for Complementary and Alternative Medicine (Barnes, Bloom, and Nahin 2008), herbal therapy or the usage of natural products other than vitamins and minerals was the most commonly used alternative medicine (18.9%)

when all use of prayer was excluded. A survey conducted in Hong Kong in 2003 reported that 40% of the subjects surveyed showed marked faith in TCM compared with Western medicine (Chan et al. 2003). In a survey of 21,923 adults in the United States, 12.8% took at least one herbal supplement (Harrison et al. 2004) and in another survey (Qato et al. 2008), 42% of respondents used dietary or nutritional supplements, with multivitamins and minerals most commonly used, followed by saw palmetto, flax, garlic, and Ginkgo, at the time of the interview.

The most common reasons for using traditional medicine are that it is more affordable, more closely corresponds to theoop patient's ideology, allays concerns about the adverse effects of chemical (synthetic) medicines, satisfies a desire for more personalized health care, and allows greater public access to health information. The major use of herbal medicines is for health promotion and therapy for chronic, as opposed to life-threatening, conditions. However, usage of traditional remedies increases when conventional medicine is ineffective in the treatment of disease, such as in advanced cancer and in the face of new infectious diseases. Furthermore, traditional medicines are widely perceived as natural and safe, that is, not toxic.

Regardless of why an individual uses it, traditional medicine provides an important health care service whether people have physical or financial access to allopathic medicine, and it is a flourishing global commercial enterprise (Engebretson 2002; Conboy). In 1990, expenditure associated with "alternative" therapy in the United States was estimated to be

US$13.7 billion. This had doubled by the year 1997, with herbal medicines growing faster than any other alternative therapy. In Australia, Canada, and the United Kingdom, annual expenditure on traditional medicine is estimated to be US$80 million, US$1 billion, and US$2.3 billion, respectively. These figures reflect the incorporation of herbal and other forms of traditional medicine into many health care systems and its inclusion in the medical training of doctors in many parts of the developed world.

- The total commercial value of the ethnobotanicals market cannot be ignored. For example, in 1995, the total turnover of nonprescription-bound herbal medicines in pharmacies was equal to almost 30% of the total turnover of non prescription-bound medicines in Germany, and in the United States, the annual retail sales of herbal products was estimated to be US$5.1 billion. In India, herbal medicine is a common practice, and about 960 plant species are used by the Indian herbal industry, of which 178 are of a high volume, exceeding 100 metric tons per year (Sahoo 2010). In China, the total value of herbal medicine manufactured in 1995 reached 17.6 billion Chinese yuan (approximately US$2.5 billion; Eisenberg et al. 1998; WHO 2001). This trend has continued, and annual revenues in Western Europe reached US$5 billion in 2003-2004 (De Smet 2005). In China, sales of herbal products totaled US$14 billion in 2005, and revenue from herbal medicines in Brazil was US$160 million in 2007 (World Health

Organization;). It is estimated that the annual worldwide market for these products approached US$60 billion (Tilburt and Kaptchuk 2008).

Currently, herbs are applied to the treatment of chronic and acute conditions and various ailments and problems such as cardiovascular disease, prostate problems, depression, inflammation, and to boost the immune system, to name but a few. In China, in 2003, traditional herbal medicines played a prominent role in the strategy to contain and treat severe acute respiratory syndrome (SARS), and in Africa, a traditional herbal medicine, the Africa flower, has been used for decades to treat wasting symptoms associated with HIV

(<u>De Smet 2005</u>; <u>Tilburt and Kaptchuk 2008</u>). Herbal medicines are also very common in Europe, with Germany and France leading in over-the-counter sales among European countries, and in most developed countries, one can find essential oils, herbal extracts, or herbal teas being sold in pharmacies with conventional drugs.

Herbs and plants can be processed and can be taken in different ways and forms, and they include the whole herb, teas, syrup, essential oils, ointments, salves, rubs, capsules, and tablets that contain a ground or powdered form of a raw herb or its dried extract. Plants and herbs extract vary in the solvent used for extraction, temperature, and extraction time, and include alcoholic extracts (tinctures), vinegars (acetic acid extracts), hot water extract (tisanes), long-term boiled extract, usually roots or bark (decoctions), and cold infusion of plants (macerates). There is no standardization, and components of an herbal extract or a product are likely to vary significantly between batches and producers.

Plants are rich in a variety of compounds. Many are secondary metabolites and include aromatic substances, most of which are phenols or their oxygen-substituted derivatives such as tannins (Hartmann 2007; Jenke-Kodama, Müller, and Dittmann 2008). Ethnobotanicals are important for pharmacological research and drug development, not only when plant constituents are used directly as therapeutic agents, but also as starting materials for the synthesis of drugs or as models for pharmacologically active compounds.

- About 200 years ago, the first pharmacologically active pure compound, morphine, was produced from opium extracted from seeds pods of the poppy *Papaver somniferum*. This discovery showed that drugs from plants can be purified and administered in precise dosages regardless of the source or age of the material (Rousseaux and Schachter 2003; Hartmann 2007). This approach was enhanced by the discovery of penicillin (<u>Li and Vederas 2009</u>). With this continued trend, products from plants and natural sources (such as fungi and marine microorganisms) or analogs inspired by them have contributed greatly to the commercial drug preparations today. Examples include antibiotics (e.g.penicillin,erythromycin); salicylic acid, a precursor of aspirin, derived from willow bark (*Salix spp.*); reserpine, an antipsychotic and antihypertensive drug from *Rauwolfia spp.*; and antimalarials such as quinine from *Cinchona* bark and lipid-lowering agents (e.g., lovastatin) from a fungus (<u>Rishton 2008</u>; <u>Schmidt et al. 2008</u>; <u>Li and Vederas 2009</u>).

Also, more than 60% of cancer therapeutics on the market or in testing are based on natural products. Of 177 drugs approved worldwide for treatment of cancer, more than 70% are based on natural products or mimetics, many of which are improved with combinatorial chemistry. It is also estimated that about 25% of the drugs prescribed worldwide are derived from plants, and 121 such active compounds are in use (Sahoo et al. 2010). Between 2005 and 2007, 13 drugs derived from natural products were approved in the United States. More than 100 natural product-based drugs are in clinical studies (Li and Vederas 2009), and of the total 252 drugs in the World Health Organization's (WHO) essential medicine list, 11% are exclusively of plant origin (Sahoo et al. 2010).

HERBAL MEDICINE AND THE AGING POPULATION

Average life expectancy at birth has increased from around 41 years in the early 1950s to approaching 80 years in many developed countries. Consequently, the percentage of elderly people (65 years and above) in our populations is increasing. The graying of our populations brings an increasing burden of chronic age-related disease and dependency. Aging is associated with a progressive decline in physiological function and an increased risk of pathological changes leading to cancer, cardiovascular disease, dementia, diabetes, osteoporosis, and so on. Lifestyle factors such as nutrition or exercise play an important role in determining the quality and duration of healthy life and in the treatment of chronic diseases (Bozzetti 2003; Benzie and Wachtel-Galor 2009, 2010). It is most likely that there is no one cause of aging, and different theories of aging have been suggested over the years. Genetic factors are undoubtedly important, but among all the metabolic theories of aging, the oxidative stress theory is the most generally supported theory (Harman 1992; Beckman and Ames 1998). This theory postulates that aging is caused by accumulation of irreversible, oxidation-induced damage (oxidative stress) resulting from the interaction of reactive oxygen species with the DNA, lipid, and protein components of cells. Antioxidants in herbs may contribute at least part of their reputed therapeutic effects (Balsano and Alisi 2009; Tang and Halliwell 2010).

With the growing popularity of herbal medicine, the "traditional" ways of identification and preparation of herbs need to be replaced with more accurate and reproducible methods so as to ensure the quality, safety, and consistency of the product. Given the market value, potential toxicity and increasing consumer demand, particularly in the sick and elderly members of our populations, regulation of production and marketing of herbal supplements and medicines require attention.

Plants, herbs, and ethnobotanicals have been used since the early days of humankind and are still used throughout the world for health promotion and treatment of disease. Plants and natural sources form the basis of today's modern medicine and contribute largely to the commercial drug preparations manufactured today. About 25% of drugs prescribed worldwide are derived from plants. Still, herbs, rather than drugs, are often used in health care. For some, herbal medicine is their preferred method of treatment. For others, herbs are used as adjunct therapy to conventional pharmaceuticals. However, in many developing societies, traditional medicine of which herbal medicine is a core part is the only system of health care available or affordable.

Chapter 3

The home herbal pantry

Creating Your Home Herbal Apothecary

The pantry and cabinets can packed tight with all manner of wonders—paper bags of carefully dried herbs, antique jars of oil infusing with aromatic plants, **blue-tinted bottles** of bioregional bitters, stoppered decanters of herbed wines, glass vials of powdered styptics, and sealed canisters of weedy tea blends. There's a spice chest in the closet, sealed buckets of **red root** and **reishi** in the pantry by a bag of rice, decoction pots stacked by the Dutch oven, and **every size of funnel** hanging next to the spatulas.

There's a variety of aesthetics, contents, and structure. But there are as many ways to envision and create an apothecary as there are herbalists. What tends to remain consistent is the **high quality** of plants, and their clearly prized status.

Organization is also a priority. Every herbalist is likely to know the frustration of searching for the one perfect formula that happens to be in an unmarked mason jar, shoved into some dusty corner for safekeeping. Such events are likely to teach us the value of storage by alphabetical order of botanical names and other such commonsense practices that seem tedious in the beginning but soon become an all-too-obvious necessity.

Whether home, clinical, or retail in nature, our herbal apothecaries exist for the storage, preservation, and distribution of botanically-based remedies. After all, the very word "apothecary" refers to a storehouse, and most any herbalist who has been about this business for any length of time will know just how .important (and how challenging) it can be to make room for their ever-expanding herbal abundance.

Purchasing Dried Herbs

The best way to assess dried plant material is to be familiar with the living plant. Barring that, I recommend reading descriptions of the scent of the plant and being familiar, if only through photos, with its appearance. This will help you know you're using the correct plant and also see how close or how far removed the dried material is from its original state.

Some herbs have specific aromatics. Certain plants, like **lemon balm**, have delicate volatile oils that are easily lost during the harvesting, drying, and storing process. I rarely expect to purchase dried lemon balm and have it be anything close to the fresh plant. However, other plants are tougher and their aromatics can survive great duress. You could toss a bag of **dried chamomile** on the side of the road in the middle of summer and come back a month later to find it still smelling distinctly of chamomile. Other plants aren't particularly aromatic, but they should still smell fresh and green, never musty.

For example, **elder flowers**, tiny as they may be, still retain many characteristics when dried properly. Expect them to be a soft ivory in color, be of recognizable form, and have the peculiar delicate scent for which they're known. **Rosehips** should still be a deep orange-red and retain their aromatic tartness if harvested at the correct time and preserved properly. Even delicate plants like *Scutellaria* have the capacity to retain their properties when dried if handled carefully. So much depends on how much moisture and light the plants have been exposed to.

Roots and seeds can be more difficult to sort out and may require that you break, scratch, or possibly heat them in order to access their aromatics. Dried plants come in a variety of colors and textures. They all change to some degree when dried, but they should generally still be **vivid in color and recognizable** when compared to the living plant.

With **bulk herbs** you can generally see and smell the quality, or lack thereof. With herbal preparations, though, it can initially be more challenging. For the most part, it helps if you know the product well before you buy, including having experienced its effects. This makes things especially difficult for beginners, many of whom have read about what an herb is like and what its actions may be, but have yet to experience it for themselves.

Making remedies is precise work. Even those employing the folkloric method (as opposed to abiding by strict measurements and proportions) must deal with detailed tasks that require both sensory and intellectual attention.

Not all preparations are created equal, but if you know the plants you're dealing with, many remedies can be fairly easy to sort out by organoleptic methods. By this, I simply mean understanding quality by using your senses. A **high-quality tincture** or **elixir** made with **fresh stinging nettles** should taste, quite distinctly, of nettle—not just boozy or like musty water. You can also tell when many products are no longer good by their scent, appearance, and other sensory keys. Plantain salve or **comfrey oil** shouldn't smell cheesy, but it often does because of the plant's water content and the tendency for some to either not wilt the plant before infusing, or to not use a **double boiler** to make sure the moisture is sufficiently removed from the fat.

Familiarity is the Key

Familiarity with plants is the key to developing an effective pharmacy. We're not merely collectors of gorgeous specimens or archivists of impersonal pharmaceutical medicines, but characters in the ancient tale of humans and plants. For longer than we have been human or had language, we have been acquainted with the ways of the green world, and we have experienced its influence on body and mind. From spit poultice to ceremonial smoke, these animals are our elders and our initiators into a deeper connection with the living land.

We've all seen the idealized apothecary photographs of gorgeous glass bottles loaded with vivid plants and spices.

Here are some recommendations to help you arrange your botanical items and guarantee that you are making the most of your herbal buddies.

THE ART OF LABELING

One of the fundamental laws of herbalism is that we should always identify our herbal mixtures and components. Here are some fundamental items I suggest including on your labels.

Name of the Herb/Preparation: The name is one of the most significant aspects of a label. You always want to know what you are taking (or serving others). When labeling preparations, I mention all of the components, so I am constantly cognizant and connected to what I'm choosing to use.

Date: This is crucial as it lets you check freshness and sift through older stuff first. Some individuals label by the date it was bought, while others label depending on when it was filled/decanted. Whatever strategy you use, just make sure you are consistent.

Uses: A fantastic method to learn more about herbs is to research them and discover their diverse applications. I discovered that it is useful to include some typical applications of the herb directly on the label so that I'm constantly linked and reminded of its supporting capabilities. As I've grown more acquainted with their usage, I've begun adding extra fascinating information so I can continue to learn and establish a stronger relationship with the plant. After all, repetition is the key to mastery.

HOW TO CHOOSE YOUR APOTHECARY JARS

Your organizing style will be greatly affected by the environment you are working in. Sure, those giant glass bottles loaded with herbs seem wonderful on Instagram, but if they produce clutter in your workstation, they may not be the ideal solution for you. Here are various jar selections that I enjoy along with their benefits and disadvantages.

Pantry Jars: As their name says, they make fantastic storage in a pantry or where you have abundant room. They are commonly used for greater volume botanicals, such as bulk teas. I love that they are airtight and keep everything extremely fresh. The negative is that they are a tad big and weighty. I don't find them to be especially beneficial for compact kitchen areas.

Cork Top Bottles: These are better for spices or ingredients that you use frequently since it's a perfect size that you can refill often. The design is lovely and provides a visually pleasant presentation. Due to the broader rim, it helps dispense bigger spices like cardamom pods or seeds. They are fantastic in compact places! The one drawback is that they don't travel nearly as well, so you may not want to take them on a picnic or camping trip.

Dual Cap Spice Bottles: These are great since you get the dual advantage of the shaker half and the open half of the lid. The style isn't as unusual as the cork caps, but they are perfect for smaller settings and give a safe method to store and transport herbs.

Stacking Spice Jars: These are great for folks who have extra vertical storage space. The stacking spice jars are a terrific way to stack herbal powders or spices you use regularly. They are constructed of acrylic, and although glass is usually preferred, this material does make them perfect travel shakers for outdoor trips.

Cobalt or Amber Glass Bottles: Generally used for herbal remedies, they come in a range of glass hues and lid options. They may be used again and over again, and typically you can swap out the lid kinds.

WHERE TO PUT YOUR APOTHECARY SUPPLIES

The presentation is a big component of your organizational approach. You should keep the following in mind while determining how you will show your herbal buddies.

Make it easy to use: The idea is to guarantee you have quick access to your preferred herbs and spices so that you're more likely to utilize and appreciate them. Some alternatives include shelves, cabinets, pantries, or even kitchen drawers.

Ensure your ingredients are simple to notice: You want to swiftly obtain what you need, or see if an unexpected ingredient option shows itself. Sometimes, inspiration leaps out at you—don't ruin the magic by concealing components under all of the other bottles! Adding layers to your cabinets can assist you in locating what you are searching for.

Maintain Freshness: Herbs keep best when they are in a dark, cold, and dry location. If you want to put your daily items on the counter or out in the open, we suggest you use smaller bottles and renew the stock more regularly. You also should not store herbs over the stove or dishwasher since these machines generate moisture and temperature changes, all of which may harm the plant material.

Pro Tips:

While having uniform jars is desirable, sometimes our finances do not enable us to attain such organization all at once. You may clean and reuse bottles as you cycle through them.

If you're having difficulties mustering the drive, print out an image of your ideal apothecary and place it near your existing storage area so you can keep your eye on the goal.

Take on the challenge in bite-size bits. Start with your first 5 or 10 most utilized herbs and work your way up. A little progress is better than no progress!

Remember that your pharmacy is a manifestation of your herbal art. It is based on all the factors that make up your specific practice. Herbalism is a lifestyle, not a phase, so don't feel forced to accomplish everything in a specific manner or all at once

Making Your Own First Aid Kit

For almost every common ailment or minor injury, there's a natural treatment that works and will give you peace of mind about treating them without scary ingredients and unnecessary preservatives. Here's how to make a first aid kit made with only all-natural ingredients for your family.

While you may not put these natural treatments into a little canvas bag or plastic box with a big red cross on it, keep them on hand for fast access when you need to treat someone in your family.

What You Need to Make a First Aid Kit

Here's what you should keep on hand:
Aloe Vera – Helpful for burns and cuts. It's easy to have a small aloe plant right outside your back door or in your kitchen window. Break off a piece and put the gel on the wound. If you don't have the plant, you can buy pure aloe vera gel.

Coconut Oil – Use as the base for salves or making tinctures. Coconut oil is antifungal and beneficial for chapped lips and dry skin. It can also be taken internally and can replace several items in your beauty routine, so choose a good quality coconut oil.

Epsom salts – Dissolve in the bath for sore muscles or to detox. For splinters, soak skin in epsom salts for 15 minutes to help remove the splinter or make it easier to remove with tweezers. We recommend buying epsom salts in bulk to save packaging waste.

Baking soda – A great bee sting remedy and everyday bug bites.

Witch **Hazel** – Keep Witch Hazel on hand for cleaning cuts and scrapes. Plus it's the most cost-effective skin toner around, and it's super useful for postpartum recovery.

Vinegar – Apple Cider Vinegar with "the mother" can be applied topically to rashes or taken internally for a variety of digestive issues.

Hydrogen Peroxide – Use for the initial cleaning of wounds, then switch to water so you don't repeatedly kill off good bacteria.

Peroxide can also help with ear infections. Place a dropper full of Hydrogen Peroxide in the ear and let rest for 15 minutes or until it stops bubbling.

Garlic oil – Garlic oil is a solid go-to for ear infections, parasites that cause diarrhea, and colds. Mullein can be added as well.

Essential oils – Every natural first aid kit should include lavender, eucalyptus, peppermint, and tea tree essential oils. These essential oils may help with most childhood ailments from headaches, minor burns and insect bites, congestion, toothaches, cold sores and digestive issues.

How to Use Your Natural First Aid Supplies

Sunburn

Bathe in cool water with Epsom salts to ease the pain. After bath, towel off and apply pure aloe vera gel to the sunburn. Few things will soothe sunburn like aloe vera gel. Keep an aloe vera plant handy in your yard and break off a leaf to rub the juice on sunburns (works great on cuts and scrapes, too).

Cuts & Scrapes

You can use Witch Hazel, vinegar or peroxide to clean the wound and aloe vera gel to help soothe the irritated skin.

Bruises

There are a few really effective <u>herbal remedies for bruising</u> you can keep in your first aid kit. The most useful one is Arnica gel.

Mosquito Bites

Few things are more irritating in the summer heat than mosquito bites. To help stop the itch, make a paste using <u>baking soda</u> and water and apply it to the bite. An alternative treatment is to crush 3 plain adult aspirin tablets and mix them with water (just a few drops) to make a paste and apply to the bite twice a day.

Bee Sting Remedy

First, make sure the person isn't allergic to bee stings. If they are, forget any home remedy and get medical attention immediately.

If there are no allergy considerations, remove the stinger by running the edge of a credit card along the welt on the skin (works

better than tweezers and you're more likely
to have a credit card handy than a pair of
tweezers anyway). Now what to put on a bee
sting? Mix 2 teaspoons of baking soda with
about a quarter teaspoon of water to make a
thick paste and apply it to the sting. Leave it
on there until the pain stops.
An alternative treatment is to mix baking
soda, vinegar, and meat tenderizer to make
a paste and apply it to the sting. Again, leave
the paste on until the pain stops.
Regardless of which paste you use, apply ice
to the sting after you remove the paste to
reduce swelling.

Poison Ivy
Pour rubbing alcohol on the affected area
and then wash it immediately with cool
water and soap to remove as much of the
plant sap as possible. Dry the skin and apply
the meat side of a banana peel on the skin to
help dry out the rash.

Swimmer's Ear Home Remedy

Who doesn't like spending time in the pool or at the beach during the summer? The downside, other than sunburn, can be swimmer's ear. First clean the ear by mixing equal parts of water, apple cider vinegar and rubbing alcohol and put one drop into each ear and let it dry. Do this twice a day.
An alternative treatment is to mix equal parts of water, white vinegar, and peroxide. Put one drop into the ear and allow it to dry. This can also be done twice a day.

DIY Essential Oil Mosquito Repellent

Why go to the trouble of putting together a natural first aid kit if you're going to keep spraying your family down with DEET every day before they go outside to keep mosquitoes at bay? Commercial insect repellents are toxic, smell awful and can cause skin rashes and breathing problems in people sensitive to the chemicals they contain. Here's an effective essential oil mosquito repellent you can feel good about using (and it smells great, too!)

In a 4-ounce glass spray bottle with a fine mist setting, combine:

- 3 ounces of distilled water
- 15 drops of Citronella essential oil
- 10 drops of Lavender essential oil
- 10 drops of Eucalyptus Globulus essential oil
- 5 drops of Lemongrass essential oil

Shake the bottle each time before you use it. Essential oils don't dissolve in water. If you don't shake the bottle before each use you run the risk of getting the concentrated oils on your skin instead of the diluted version, and you could have some skin irritation as a result.

Mist your skin and clothing with the mixture and reapply it as needed.

The great thing about natural first aid treatments is that you will have most of these items in your kitchen pantry or bathroom medicine cabinet. The key is knowing how to use them to treat common illnesses and injuries and having them in a place where you can get to them quickly when you need them.

Many people are surprised to find those little tins and bottles of spices in your kitchen cabinet can also be used in a pinch for natural first aid

It's simple to take down a tin of a spice, put some in your hand, add a little carrier oil or purified water and make a quick poultice. You can also use them to make a quick medicinal tea. As always, make sure they are organically grown and pure.

Here are a few herbs and spices you can use for natural first aid:

Basil – good for relieving headaches because it has antispasmodic properties. It will also help with nervous indigestion and stress induced insomnia.

Cardamom – good for clearing the lungs. You can use it in a tea.

Chives – works in a way very similar to garlic but it's not as strong. Very good for indigestion and to boost the respiratory system. If you find you have a problem with garlic, try chives instead.

Cinnamon – clears congestion, stimulates circulation and has strong antiseptic qualities.

Cloves – a great pain killing herb used extensively for toothaches but it can also be used to relieve nausea.

Dill – excellent for colic and indigestion. You can give it in a tea or a tincture.

Ginger – excellent for nausea, congestion, sore throats, colds and flu.

Rosemary – great for congestion and for digestive problems.

Sage – a great liver tonic and helps with digestion after a meal of fatty or greasy food. It also has antiseptic properties so use it for colds, flu and sore throats.

Thyme – excellent for coughs, colds, sore throats and giving the immune system a boost.

Turmeric – one of the absolute best spices for the immune system and has strong anti-tumor and antibiotic properties. You can also apply it topically in a paste or poultice for burns, cuts, scrapes and bruises.

Chapter 4

Herbal First Aid kit

Emergency preparation doesn't only have to come in the shape of a shop-purchased case. You may start by working with what you can acquire, If you live someplace hot, you'll want to protect yourself against dehydration and other sun-related ailments. If mosquitoes are abuzz near you, scroll down for some vital post-bite treatment.

Here are the top treatments our herbalists suggest you carry or have access to at all times,

*There are various variations as to how to produce the medications below. Depending on your requirements, and desire it may vary anywhere from tea, tinctures (alcohol-based extracts), glycerinates (vegetable glycerin-based extracts), salves, and much more.

CALENDULA

Internal Use: Antiviral, vulnerary, and anti-inflammatory

External Use: A skin super tonic used for wounds, scrapes, burns, and rashes

CALIFORNIA POPPY

Internal Use: Pain reliever, mild sedative

External Use: Topical analgesic

CHILCUAGUE

Internal Use: The "golden root" may defend against parasites, reduce tooth and muscular aches, and inhibit sore throat and fungal infections like canker sores

External Use: Treats herpes blisters, lessens bug bite pain and itching

COMFREY

Internal Use: For brief periods of time, it may aid with bone repair.

External Use: Wounds, ulcers, sprains, strains, and discomfort.

ECHINACEA

Internal Use: Anti-viral, anti-microbial, antiseptic, wound healing + useful after bites, stings, and allergies, in addition to food poisoning/bacterial infection

ELDERBERRY

Internal Use: Prevents and cures colds and upper respiratory illnesses

CHAMOMILE

Internal: Digestive relaxant, helpful for GI problems, indigestion, diarrhea, anorexia, motion sickness, and nausea. Assists youngsters with colic, fevers, and coughing.

External: Antiseptic, antibacterial, anti-fungal.

GOLDEN SEAL

Internal Use: Antibiotic, helps fight infections, and may assist with digestive stress such as traveler's diarrhea

External Use: Apply to cuts or wounds to stop bleeding; tea may be used as an eyewash to alleviate eye irritation *Be careful to obtain Golden Seal exclusively from farms that properly and ethically produce it. Do not promote unethical wildcrafting since it's in extinction.

KRATOM

Internal + External Use: One of the finest pain relievers, which may be used as a topical or internal analgesic *Avoid excessive usage, and utilize wisely.

NETTLE

Internal Use: Daily multivitamin and mineralizer utilized for repair and strength; especially beneficial for the womb during menstruation, pregnancy, and more.

PLANTAIN

InternalUse: Anti-inflammatory
frequently used to alleviate coughs,
mucus, and membrane irritation

External Use: A poultice may be eaten (or
the leaf crushed) to apply to bites, stings,
burns, wounds, and scrapes

PEPPERMINT

Internal Use: Relieves headaches, and
stomach discomfort, and may help break a
fever

External Use: Use a tea bag or compress to
reduce inflammation, heat, or itching

YARROW

Internal Use: Fights infection, increases
perspiration, and decreases fever; also
enhances circulation and blood flow and
soothes digestive tension and cramps

External Use: A genuine heal-all, great for wounds (a coagulant), antiseptic, antimicrobial, antibacterial, and antifungal; topically used to stop bleeding, cure cuts, scrapes, burns, and rashes or for varicose veins/rheumatic joints

WHITE WILLOW

Internal Use: The "origin of aspirin" is a potent anti-inflammatory, pain reliever, and antipyretic to keep on hand at all times

JARGON SACHA

Internal Use: Antivenom,antiviral, anti-inflammatory, and antispasmodic. Used as mashed raw root in water, or as a decoction.

External Use: Applied as a poultice topically on snake bites and wounds.

MULUNGU

Internal Use: Nervine, a hypnotic sedative, reduces hysteria from trauma or shock. Must be administered as a decoction or extract to obtain its full benefits

Simple and Effective Herbal Home Remedies

Soothe aches, bruises, stings and more with these DIY cures.

Avocado smoothie

GOOD FOR: Constipation

Avocados contain magnesium, a mineral that acts as a laxative by drawing water into the intestinal tract to keep things moving. For a stomach-soothing smoothie, blend ½ avocado, ½ cup raspberries, ½ cup unsweetened almond milk and a handful of ice.

Blueberry water

GOOD FOR: Urinary tract infections

Just like cranberries, blueberries contain substances that prevent bacteria from sticking in your bladder. To ward off UTIs, combine 1 part unsweetened blueberry juice with 2 parts water and sip daily.

Carrot Compress

GOOD FOR: Insect bites and stings

A carrot compress can help reduce inflammation and dry out insect bites and stings to take out the itch. Finely grate a carrot and wrap the pulp in a thin paper towel or cheesecloth. Place on swelling for 20 minutes, store in the refrigerator and repeat four times in 24 hours.

Deep breathing

GOOD FOR: Hot flashes

When you're in the throes of a hot flash, deep breathing can help stop it in its tracks by calming your nervous system quickly. Just take a deep breath in for a count of four, feeling your belly rise, then breathe out slowly and fully for a count of four. Repeat this sequence four more times in succession.

Epsom salts

GOOD FOR: Dry, cracked skin

Smooth your elbows and heels with this inexpensive at-home treatment: Mix ½ cup Epsom salt with ½ cup water to make a paste. Exfoliate by gently massaging into rough areas, then rinsing with water.

Green tea

GOOD FOR: Colds

Viruses that cause the sniffles often start in the back of your mouth and throat. Stop them from spreading with a cleansing gargle. At the first sign of symptoms, combine 1 tsp salt with 2 cups strong green tea. Stir and refrigerate. Gargle twice daily, using ½ cup at a time.

Honey

GOOD FOR: Pimples

Wake up with a blemish? Dab a bit of honey on it in the morning. (You can leave it on all day, even under your makeup.) Honey works as an antiseptic to stop the growth of bacteria that can cause breakouts.

Ice pack

GOOD FOR: Bruises

Bumps can leave an ugly mark, but applying ice to the area several times a day helps decrease the pain and discoloration. For a

DIY ice pack, mix 1 part rubbing alcohol with 3 parts water in a resealable bag and freeze. (The solution will remain slushy, so you can mold the bag around the bruise.)

Kneading massage

GOOD FOR: Relieving anxiety

If you're feeling stressed, put pressure on the point located between your thumb and index finger. (Use the opposite thumb and forefinger to squeeze and release the muscle for 30 seconds.)

Licorice root

GOOD FOR: Cold sores

Licorice root can kill the viruses that cause herpes around your mouth. Steep a licorice tea bag in warm water for 30 to 60 seconds, then apply for 3 to 5 minutes. Repeat daily until sores subside.

Cheese

GOOD FOR: Leg cramps

A charley horse can disrupt sleep, so snack on 1 oz lowfat cheese and a few walnuts an hour before bed. Cheese has magnesium and calcium, which relax your muscles and nervous system, while the walnuts contain melatonin, a sleep-promoting brain chemical. Eat dairy to calm your body before you hit the sheets.

Olives

GOOD FOR: Nausea

Olives contain tannins, which are chemicals that help slow down the excessive production of saliva (one of the first symptoms of motion sickness). Eat a few green or black olives as soon as you start to feel woozy.

Pick-Me-Up Shower

GOOD FOR: A mood booster

Try a "contrast shower." Switching from hot to cold water is stimulating, and experts say it can help relieve gloominess by increasing circulation. Shower in warm water for 3 minutes, then quickly switch to chilly for 30 seconds. Repeat that cycle three times, ending on cold.

Quick Stroll

GOOD FOR: A brain jolt

When you're feeling mentally tired, go for a brisk 5-minute walk. Moving your muscles immediately increases the activity in your brain so you feel more awake and alert.

Refreshing rinse

GOOD FOR: Bad breath

To battle halitosis and whiten teeth, combine a cup of water with 1 tsp baking soda, swish around in your mouth, then spit out. The baking soda helps to fight smelly bacteria and combats dry mouth.

Smart stretch

GOOD FOR: Headaches

Tension headaches are often caused by sitting hunched over a computer screen. (The position tightens muscles in the front of your neck and chest.) Do this simple move to undo the damage: Stand up and put your hands on hips. Roll head back so you're staring at the ceiling as you arch your back slightly.

Tropical fruit

GOOD FOR: Pain relief

Whip up a drink that's filled with strong ingredients to alleviate inflammation and promote blood flow to hasten recovery. Combine ½ oz bottled lemon juice with ½ oz ginger juice with 1 oz pineapple juice and a pinch each of cayenne pepper and turmeric. Drink anytime you have painful muscles.

High blood pressure therapy

A fantastic natural cure for high blood pressure is drinking blueberry juice or garlic water regularly. In addition, many plants put in teas, such as hibiscus tea or olive leaf tea, seem to have great antihypertensive qualities which assist in lowering blood pressure.

Learn about natural therapies and lifestyle adjustments you may use to supplement your high blood pressure therapy.

1. Garlic water

Garlic water is a natural technique to manage blood pressure since it encourages the synthesis of nitric oxide. This is a gas with a high vasodilation effect, which promotes blood circulation and relieves strain on the heart.

In addition, garlic is also beneficial for preserving cardiovascular health, as it contains remarkable antioxidant capabilities that protect the blood vessels.

One approach to ingesting garlic is by infusing it in water and sipping it throughout the day.

Ingredients

1 clove of raw garlic, peeled and crushed; 3.4 oz (100 ml) of water.

Preparation method

Place the garlic clove in a cup of water and let it soak for six to eight hours (or overnight). After this time, consume it before breakfast on an empty stomach. If you like, you may also double the ingredients above to have numerous servings of this infusion

You may also take garlic as a part of your meals throughout the day, since it may be more fun to eat garlic than to drink it. A nice option is to add some peeled cloves to your olive oil for a garlic-infused alternative (this will enable you to benefit from the garlic characteristics every time you drink olive oil).

2. Reduce salt consumption

Sodium, which is a crucial component of salt, has the power to attract water into your blood vessels, which increases the amount of circulating blood. This raises the pressure inside your blood vessels, which in turn leads to a rise in blood pressure. To avoid hypertension, you should eat fewer than 2300 mg of salt each day.

Those who have previously been diagnosed with hypertension should lower their salt consumption to 1500 mg - 2300 mg per day.

3. Olive leaf tea

Just like garlic, olive tree leaves are one of the finest natural therapies for high blood pressure. They contain polyphenols that control blood pressure, without the danger of inducing hypotension, even if ingested in excess.

In addition, they also have a mild soothing and relaxing impact, which helps to regulate anxiety symptoms.

Ingredients

2 tablespoons of ground olive leaves; 16.9 oz (500 ml) of boiling water.

Preparation method

Place the olive leaves in a kettle with boiling water and let the leaves soak for five to ten minutes. Then filter the mixture using a mesh strainer and let it cool down. You may drink three to four cups of tea throughout the day.

In addition to the tea, there is also an olive leaf extract that can be obtained in shops in the form of capsules. Capsules may be taken in quantities of 500 mg, twice a day after meals.

4. Regular exercise

Exercise is a fantastic method to not only build your complete body but also your heart. A powerful heart may operate more effectively to pump blood, which might affect high blood pressure levels. Patients wanting to avoid hypertension or lower raised blood pressure levels should attempt to exercise 4 times per week for 30 to 60 minutes. Activities should be of moderate intensity and might include walking, running, cycling, or swimming. Studies demonstrate that greater intensity exercise is not more helpful for the prevention or control of hypertension in comparison to moderate intensity.

5. Blueberry juice

In addition to being a good source of antioxidants, which fight illnesses like cancer and prevent aging, blueberries can help reduce blood pressure, particularly when ingested frequently.

The benefits of blueberries are particularly noticeable in those with high cardiovascular risk, such as those who are obese or those who have metabolic syndrome. Therefore, blueberry juice may be used as a natural supplement to any high blood pressure medication provided by the doctor.

Ingredients

1 cup of fresh blueberries; ½ cup of water; Juice squeezed from ½ lemon.

Preparation method

Place all the ingredients in a blender and mix until smooth. You may drink this juice once or twice a day.

6. Healthy body weight

Maintaining a healthy body weight and waist size are connected with decreased risk for cardiovascular disease. Patients are encouraged to maintain their BMI between 18 and 24 to avoid or cure hypertension. Women should try to maintain their waist circumference below 88 cm, while males should be below 102 cm.

7. Hibiscus tea

Hibiscus is a plant that is quite popular amongst individuals who wish to lose weight, yet this plant may also assist in decreasing blood pressure. This is due to its high content of anthocyanins, which are flavonoids that assist control of blood pressure.

To achieve optimum blood pressure results, it is advisable to utilize the flower calyxes with deeper hues. The calyxes are the structures that link the stem to the petals. The darker the hibiscus blossoms are, the larger the concentration of anthocyanins and the better the action against high blood pressure.

Ingredients 1 - 2 grams of hibiscus calyxes; 1 cup of boiling water.

Preparation method

Place the hibiscus calyxes in the heated water and let them soak for five to ten minutes. Then filter the mixture with a mesh screen and drink this tea once to twice a day, making sure you leave at least eight hours between each cup of tea.

Even though there are no studies that verify this yet, hibiscus may be poisonous over a daily intake of six grams. Therefore, it is suggested that you do not take more than the dosage mentioned above.

Hibiscus tea may have a bitter flavor, so if required, you may add a teaspoon of stevia or honey to the concoction.

8. Limit alcohol intake

Alcohol may alter the way your heart operates by making it beat faster. Consistent, excessive alcohol usage may elevate blood pressure over time and increase your overall risk for cardiovascular disease. For this reason, healthy individuals are recommended to restrict their alcohol consumption to 2 drinks per day. Men should not exceed 14 drinks in a week, while women should not exceed 9 drinks in a week.

9. Mangaba tea

Another wonderful natural cure for high blood pressure is eating a fruit called mangaba or drinking a mangaba bark tea. This plant helps with vasodilation, decreasing blood pressure.

Ingredients

2 teaspoons of magaba bark; 16.9 oz (500 ml) of boiling water.

Preparation method

Add the bark to the boiling water and let the mixture soak for a few minutes. Cover the saucepan, let the tea cool down, and then filter. You may drink two to three glasses every day.

10. Healthy diet

Healthy diet is generally recommended for the prevention and management of hypertension in adults. This diet comprises the reduction of saturated fat and cholesterol and highlights the significance of fruits, vegetables, and low-fat dairy products in regular meals. Patients should attempt to consume dietary and soluble fiber, whole grains, and protein from plant sources in every meal.

Patients who have been diagnosed with high blood pressure may be recommended to restrict their potassium consumption since higher potassium levels might contribute to high blood pressure.

11. Horsetail tea

Horsetail tea is a good natural diuretic that promotes the production of urine and removes extra fluid from the body. It may be a fantastic tea for decreasing blood pressure in persons who have a lot of fluid retention, since the extra water in the body produces greater stress on the heart, which can increase hypertension.

Despite its advantages, this tea should only be consumed rarely, for instance, when it is tougher to manage blood pressure with conventional techniques and when there is a lot of fluid retention. This tea must not be consumed for more than one week, since it also leads to the evacuation of vital minerals via the urine.

Ingredients

2 to 3 teaspoons of dried horsetail leaves; 16.9 oz (500 ml) of boiling water.

Preparation method

Place the horsetail leaves in the boiling water and let the mixture settle for five to ten minutes. Then drain the mixture and sip the tea while it is warm. This tea may be taken two to three times a day.

12. Valerian tea

Valerian roots offer strong soothing and relaxing effects that assist in enhancing blood circulation. In addition, valerian tea works directly on the GABA neurotransmitter, which may aid people who suffer from regular anxiety episodes and have high blood pressure as a consequence.

Ingredients

5 grams of dried valerian root; 1 cup of boiling water.

Preparation method

Place the valerian roots in a cup of boiling water and let the mixture soak for five to ten minutes. Then filter with a mesh screen and drink two to three times a day. In some individuals, valerian tea might promote tiredness throughout the day. If you suffer any sleepiness, it should only be taken at night.

13.Stress management

Some patients may benefit from relaxation techniques if stress or anxiety plays a role in elevated blood pressure readings. Individualized cognitive behavioral therapies are found to be effective, as well as meditation, yoga or acupuncture.

Chapter 5

Some Plants and their botanical names for common ailments.

E. guineensis Jacq (Arecaceae), popularly known as oil palm is a monocotyledonous plant which belongs to the coccoid group of palms. It grows up to 15 m high with a lifetime of over 100 years and occurs throughout the tropical rainforest belt of West Africa. _E. guineensis_ is commonly used for treating gonorrhea, rheumatism, headache, wounds . An _in vitro_ anti-plasmodial assay revealed that, the ethanolic extract of _E. guineensis_ leaves has potent antimalarial activity.

Phyllanthus emblica
P. emblica. of the family Euphorbiaceae is a deciduous medium-sized plant (10–18 m high), native to tropical south eastern Asia and widely distributed in most subtropical and tropical countries. It is commonly

known as Indian gooseberry, rich in vitamin C, minerals and amino acids which helps to build up lost vitality and vigor. Various parts of the plant is used traditionally for the treatment of diarrhea, inflammation, diabetes, jaundice, cough, asthma, peptic ulcer, skin diseases, leprosy, intermittent fevers, headache, anemia, dizziness, snakebite and scorpion-sting.

Syzygium aromaticum

S. aromaticum (L.) Merril. & Perry, syn. *Eugenia caryophyllata*, an ancient and valuable spice is a member of the family Myrtaceae and is commonly known as clove. It is mostly used as a spice to flavor all kinds of foods and has other medicinal values including anthelmintic, anti-asthma and other allergic disorders, anti-inflammatory, antioxidant, antiviral and anti-parasitic properties.

Casearia sylvestris

C. sylvestris is an evergreen shrub or small tree with long, slender branches and a very dense globose crown. Usually 4–6 m tall, but can grow up to 20 m high, with wide distribution throughout South America. It has been employed in traditional medicine for treating snake bites, wounds, inflammation, fevers, gastric ulcers and diarrhea.

Cupania vernalis

C. vernalis Cambess. (Sapindaceae) is a semi-deciduous tree with elongated and dense crown, which can grow up to 10–22 m tall. It can be found in almost all forest formations in Brazil, South America, Argentina, Uruguay, Paraguay and Bolivia. The tree serves as source of tannins and wood locally, and in traditional medicine as diuretic, stimulant, expectorant, natural surfactant, sedative and for treating stomach-ache and dermatitis. The hexane and ethanol leaf extracts showed active antimalarial activity against chloroquine-resistance

Xylopia emarginata

X. emarginata Mart. is a species of plant in the Annonaceae family. It is native to Cerrado vegetation in Brazil. It is an evergreen tree with a very narrow, almost columnar crown which can grow up to 10–20 m tall and 30–40 cm in diameter. It usually grows in large clusters, forming a homogeneous mass. It is a species characteristic of swamp forest, and does not grow in the driest places. It is used as a condiment in food, a carminative and aphrodisiac in traditional medicine.

Xylopia *aromatic*

X. aromatica (Lam.) Mart. belongs to the family Annonaceae and the accepted name is *X. xylopioides*. It is a medium-sized tree with long, hanging branches that can make the crown look like a Christmas tree. Leaves are alternate, narrow, pointed, in a flat plane and arranged regularly along the branches. It is a common roadside and farmland species of the Pacific slope, not in the forest. The root wood and root bark hexane extracts demonstrated an *in vitro* antimalarial activity against chloroquine-resistance (FcB1/Colombia) strains of *P. falciparum*

Aspidosperma macrocarpon

A. macrocarpon Mart. (Apocynaceae) is a deciduous tree with an open crown growing up to 3–25 m tall and 25-35 cm in diameter. Traditionally, it is employed in the treatment of fever .

Azadirachta indica

A. indica A. Juss is commonly known as neem tree or Indian lilac and belongs to the mahogany family Meliaceae. It is an evergreen, fast-growing tree that can reach a height of 15–20 m with few of them growing up to 35–40 m, but in severe drought it may shed most of its leaves or nearly all leaves. It is typically grown in tropical and semi-tropical regions. Neem is effective against certain fungi that infect humans and hence used to treat skin diseases like eczema, psoriasis .

Maytenus senegalensis

M. senegalensis Lam. Exell which belongs to the family Celastraceae is an African shrubs or trees widely distributed throughout Central and South America, Southeast Asia, Micronesia and Australasia, the Indian Ocean and Africa, growing up to 15 m high with spines up to 7 cm long. Traditionally, it is an anti-inflammatory herbal drug and is useful in treating toothaches. The stem bark methanol extract showed anti-plasmodial activity.

Medicinal plants with demonstrated activity against *Vibrio cholera*

Cholera is an acute intestinal disease caused by a facultative anaerobic, Gram-negative, comma-shaped rod bacterium, known as *V. cholerae*. Cholera is a life threatening disease transmitted by the fecal-oral route. The organisms adhere to and colonize the small bowel within a short incubation period, where they secrete cholera enterotoxin leading to severe and watery diarrhea accompanied with vomiting, dehydration and eventually death if not treated promptly. Various antibiotics have been effective for the treatment of cholera; however, the worldwide problem of microbial resistance to existing antimicrobial medicines has led to most antibiotic failure.

Researchers are therefore shifting their focus to natural products, especially medicinal plant, with effective antimicrobial properties. Some medicinal plants with potent anti-cholera activity are reviewed below.

Terminalia chebula

T. chebula Retz. (Combretaceae) commonly known as black or chebulic myrobalan is a medium to large deciduous tree growing up to 30 m tall, with a trunk of 1 m in diameter.

It leaves are oval, alternate to subopposite in arrangement and is a native to South Asia, from India and Nepal east to southwest China, Sri Lanka, Malaysia and Vietnam. Traditionally, it has been used for treatment of indigestion, diarrhea and diabetes .
The plant extract used to treat Cholera worked effectively against the strains of *V. cholera* the causative agent. The methanol fruit extract of *T. chebula* had strong bactericidal activity

Syzygium cumini

S. cumini known as Jam is an evergreen tropical tree, native to the Indian Subcontinent, adjoining regions of Southeast Asia, China and Queensland. It Grows up to 30 m and can live more than 100 years, with a dense foliage which provides shade and is grown just for its ornamental value. The leaves are pinkish when young, and changes to dark green with a yellow midrib as they mature. The seeds have traditionally been used to treat diarrhea, dysentery, piles, indigestion and diabetes. *S. cumini* methanol seed extract exhibited a bactericidal anti-cholera activity against multi-drug resistance strains of *V. cholerae*

Saraca indica

S. indica commonly known as Asoka-tree or Ashok is a plant belonging to the Detarioideae subfamily of the Fabaceae family. Asoka tree is an evergreen tree with a spreading crown which can grow up to 24 m tall and 34 cm in diameter. The original plant specimen came from Java. Some traditional uses of the plant include treatment of dyspepsia, fever, burning sensation, colic, ulcers, menorrhagia, leucorrhoea, pimples. S. *indica* evoked strong bactericidal activity against different strains of multi-drug resistance *V. cholera*.

Butea monosperma

B. monosperma (Papilionaceae) is a native to tropical and sub-tropical parts of the

Indian Subcontinent and Southeast Asia, ranging across India, Bangladesh, Nepal, Sri Lanka, Myanmar, Thailand, Laos, Cambodia, Vietnam, Malaysia and western Indonesia. Common names include flame-of-the-forest and bastard teak. It is a medium-sized dry season-deciduous tree, growing to 15 m tall. Leaves are pinnate, with (8–16 cm) petiole and three leaflets of 10–20 cm long. Its flowers are used in traditional medicine for the treatment of ulcer, inflammation, hepatic disorder and eye diseases.The methanol flower extract showed anti-cholera activity

Euphorbia serpens

E. serpens Kunth is a member of the Euphorbiaceae family. It is native to South America but it can be found on most continents as an introduced species and often a weed. This is an annual herb forming a mat of prostrate stems. Purified bioactive fraction of aqueous extract of *E. serpens* exhibited an anti-Vibrio activity

Ocimum basilicum

O. basilicum can be found in Tropical Asia.
It is a perennial growing up to 0.5 m tall and
by 0.3 m in diameter. Medicinally it is used
for the treatment of fever, colds, influenza,
poor digestion, nausea, abdominal cramps,
gastro-enteritis, migraine, insomnia,
depression and exhaustion. The methanol
whole plant extract exhibited a bactericidal
activity against *V. cholera* .

Lawsonia inermis

L. inermis Linn. (Apocynaceae) commonly
known in India as Henna is a flowering
plant and the sole species of the genus
Lawsonia. It is a tall shrub or small tree,
standing 1.8–7.6 m tall, glabrous and
multi-branched, with spine-tipped
branchlets. The henna plant is native to
northern Africa, western and southern Asia,
northern Australia, and thrives well in
semi-arid zones and tropical areas. It is
useful medicinally for burning sensation,

leprosy, skin diseases, amenorrhoea, and dysmenorrhea and as abortifacient.

Cinnamomum verum

C. verum, (formerly *C. zeylanicum*) of the family Lauraceae, commonly known as cinnamon tree is an evergreen small tropical plant native to Sri Lanka, it is also cultivated in Madagascar and Seychelles on commercial scale. Its anti-tuberculosis activity reported by Sivakumar and Jayaraman, revealed that, the aqueous and ethanolic extracts of the bark of *C. verum* exhibited anti-mycobacterial activity

Medicinal plants with demonstrated activity against pneumonia

Pneumonia is a respiratory tract infection characterized by the inflammation of one or both lungs as a results of the accumulation of pus in the alveoli. Pneumonia which can be caused by bacteria, viruses or fungi can be mild, severe or life threatening. Bacterial pneumonia can be caused by *Streptococcus pneumoniae* which is the commonest cause, *Staphylococcus aureus, Moraxella catarrhalis, Klebsiella pneumoniae, Haemophilus influenza, Chlamydophila pneumonia* and *Legionella pneumophila. Pneumocystis jirovecii pneumonia* (PCP) is a fungal pneumonia commonly found in immuno compromised patients. Viral pneumonia can also be caused by adenovirus, Varicella zoster, Influenza virus and respiratory syncytial virus . Traditionally, medicinal plants have been employed for treating pneumonia and hence the need to prove, scientifically, their folkloric uses. Researchers have investigated such plant, and below is a review on some of the reported plants with demonstrated activity.

Echinops adenocaulos

In Ethiopian herbal medicine, members of the genus *Echinops* from family Asteraceae are used for the treatment of diarrhea, intestinal worm infestation, hemorrhoids, migraine and different forms of infections. Zamzam water extract of *E. adenocaulos* demonstrated an antibacterial activity against multidrug resistance *S. pneumoniae* with a minimum inhibitory concentration (MIC) of 0.781 mg/mL.

Verbascum fruticulosum

Various species of *Verbascum*, of the family Scrophulariaceae, have been used to treat pulmonary diseases in traditional medicine as a results of its antibacterial activity against *Klebsiella pneumonia* and *Staphylococcus aureus. The in vitro* antimicrobial activity of aqueous extract of *V. fruticulosum* against multidrug resistant clinical isolate of *S. pneumoniae* showed a high antibacterial activity.

Parietaria judaica

P. judaica commonly known as pellitory of wall from family Urticaceae has been valued for its use as a diuretic, balm for wounds and burns and also as a soother for chronic cough in herbal medicine.

Medicinal plants with demonstrated anti-asthmatic activity

Asthma is a complex inflammatory disease and congestive respiratory disorder brought about by airway narrowing. It symptoms may include episodic wheezing, cough and chest tightness resulting in airflow block. It leads to changes in the levels of eosinophils, mast cells, lymphocytes, cytokines and other inflammatory cell products. There is increased prevalence worldwide especially in industrialized countries and among children with increased morbidity and mortality rate. Medicinal plants have been screened for properties that enhance their activity as anti-asthmatic agents, since current medications have adverse side effects. Few of such plants with demonstrated activity are reviewed below.

Curcuma longa

C. longa L. is a rhizomatous herbaceous perennial flowering plant of the ginger family, Zingiberaceae. It is native to the Indian subcontinent and Southeast Asia, and requires temperatures between 20 and 30°C and a considerable amount of annual rainfall to thrive. Methanolic extracts (curcumin-II at 200 mg/kg and curcumin-I at 100 mg/kg) of the finger rhizomes of *C. longa* reduced significantly ($P < 0.01$) estimated white blood cells count in ovalbumin (OVA) sensitized Wistar rat models for both long and short term. At a higher dosage, curcumin-II (200 mg/kg) tends to protect intact mast cells from degranulation. This suggests that curcumin can be used as complementary medicine in the treatment of Asthma.

Aerva lanata

A. lanata is a perennial herb, frequently becoming more or less woody at the base. The stems can be erect to prostrate, sometimes scrambling or climbing into other plants for support. It is widespread in the tropics and subtropics of Africa through Asia to the Philippines and New Guinea. It is used traditionally for treating cough, sore throat, indigestion, wounds, and diabetics and as a vermifuge for children.

Cynodon dactylon

C. dactylon (L.) Pers, of the family Poaceae is a short-lived, prostrate, perennial grass. It is widely naturalized in the temperate to tropical zones of Europe, Africa, Asia, the Pacific and the Americas. Its habitat is along roadsides and in exposed rocky or sandy sites. It use in traditional medicine to stop bleeding in minor injuries, for weak vision and eye disorders, piles, asthma, tumors among others.

Piper betle

P. betle commonly referred to as Betel pepper, is an evergreen climbing shrub producing woody stems, 5–20 m long, and distributed in Southeast Asia—probably originally from Malaysia. It is traditionally used to cure cough, cold, pruritis, asthma and rheumatism.

Lepidium sativum

L. sativum also referred to as Garden cress is a profusely-branched, erect, annual plant growing up to 80 cm tall. It commonly grown in many regions of Saudi Arabia and the Eastern Province. The seeds are used to cure bronchitis, asthma, cough, and useful as abortifacient, antibacterial, aphrodisiac, diuretic, expectorant, gastrointestinal stimulant, gastroprotective, laxative and stomachic.

Conclusion

All the plants reviewed exhibited potent activity confirming their various traditional uses and their ability to treat prevalent diseases.

www.ingramcontent.com/pod-product-compliance
Lightning Source LLC
Chambersburg PA
CBHW070817260726
48660CB00005B/1882